In Defense of the Nurse Practitioner
Removing Barriers to Practice
Ian A. Lane

Correspondence may be addressed to: ianlane88@gmail.com

Keywords: Advanced Practice Nurse; Registered Nurse; Nurse Practitioner; Medical Doctor; Physician; Osteopathic Physician; Physician Assistant; Primary Care Provider

Background

Since 1965, after the start of the first pediatric nurse practitioner program in the United States,[1] a heated debate has erupted, and rages on, between medical doctors and nurse practitioners. On one side of the debate, nurse practitioners are concerned primarily with practicing to the full extent of their license, without being barred from doing so by another health profession. On the other hand, physicians, as evidenced by the formal position statements issued by the American Medical Association (AMA) and its auspices,[2-3] generally seem to believe that nurse practitioners wish to replace physicians, and, due to their apparently substandard training, would be a blight to patient safety, should their limited scope of practice be expanded further. This kind of misunderstanding and misrepresentation of perspectives is arguably the biggest problem in this discussion.

A Misinformed Debate

A popular argument against the autonomous nurse practitioner, frequently cited by various extensions of the medical establishment, is actually a straw man. That nurse practitioners want independent clinical practice, totally cut off from any interprofessional collaboration is not the same as saying that nurse practitioners want the freedom to practice with the clinical autonomy that reflects their level of education and training, without explicit medical oversight. Nurse practitioners are well aware that they are not physicians, nor do they wish to be. That is precisely why they chose to become nurses, instead. That is to say that many nurses are intelligent enough to have gone to medical school, but chose differently; perhaps for philosophical reasons, or quality-of-life reasons. Regardless of one's rationale for making such a personal decision, to assume that they merely could not succeed in medicine and therefore settled for nursing is an insult to the profession.

Another conflation is the idea that, because nurse practitioners are seeking greater autonomy and professional responsibility, they will inevitably lobby to perform solo surgeries and interpret PET scans. This is a good example of the Slippery Slope fallacy. Nurse practitioners do not seek an expanded scope of practice, per se. They merely seek to dissolve those blockades the medical establishment has imposed on their ability to practice uniformly across all fifty states, so they may have more professional consistency, and finally be able to practice to the full extent of their license regardless of where they choose to live and work.

As it stands, a nurse practitioner working in rural New York could move to south Florida with his or her family and have a completely different set of professional guidelines, simply because that state's laws may lack consistency with other states. It seems obvious that the legal practice rights for nurse practitioners in the United States ought to be consistent, across all state lines; perhaps even regulated on a federal level, rather than on a state level, as currently practiced. If a provider is educated and trained to perform a certain set of clinical functions in one part of the country, and then moves his or her practice to another part, it is unreasonable to limit this person's ability to maintain the same set of functions they had been previously performing, assuming the quality of said performance was of demonstrably high quality.

As one considers the interference of the medical establishment with the advancement of the nursing profession, it begs the question: If a provider is educated and trained to perform a specific set of tasks under one model of care, what gives another organization the right to limit said professionals' ability to practice to that limit? At this time, it seems to be based on fear. Fear that nurses are a conniving group, looking to subversively trample all over medicine's prestigious rose garden. This could not be further from the truth, and is based precisely on those cognitive fallacies previously mentioned. It is time we move beyond these illogical constructs and think critically and clearly, with a utilitarian ethic in mind, for the good of all involved.

Independence or Autonomy?

It is important to recognize that, although the colloquial definitions of the words *autonomous* and *independent* are synonymous, they do not innately mean the same thing in health care. The concept of the nurse practitioner unjustifiably fighting to secure for themselves clinical freedom, independent of the integration of other professional opinions, is integral to the narrative their opponents use when arguing this topic. Where clinical independence in postmodern medicine is considered the diagnosis and treatment of any condition that presents to the clinic, without unsolicited input from any other professional, autonomy has embraced a different connotation. Autonomous providers craft appropriate diagnoses and treatment plans for their patients, without the explicit oversight of other practitioners who are expected to micromanage their caseload. This distinction is imperative, since the idea of true clinical independence has never existed for anyone, doctors or nurses alike.

A prime example is the newfound fight for clinical autonomy brought forth by professionals in the physical therapy community.[4] As they are arguably the resident experts in non-operative neuro-musculoskeletal therapies, musculoskeletal pain and movement disorders, many physical therapists believe they ought to be given the right to see patients as front-line providers, without patients' requiring a referral from their primary care providers. In the PT world, since these therapists have always lingered on the outside, as an "allied health" provider, never quite being offered an appropriate place at the table, this is being referred to as direct access care. The multitude of new providers now invested in this movement, along with the American Physical Therapy Association (APTA), realize that, even though physical therapists now require a doctoral degree to enter into clinical practice, they are not trained in the diagnosis and management of disease, per se, and so are not qualified to handle systemic illness, or concerns related to other body systems. In fact, they do not assess pathology, at all. They are experts in human movement systems and neuro-musculoskeletal dysfunction. However, one could argue that, as compared to the average primary care physician, a doctor of physical therapy will have amassed far more practice hours dealing with these organ systems, and are typically much more proficient at patient assessment in this area. Not to mention, many physical therapy programs have added differential diagnosis coursework to their doctoral curricula to prepare these graduates to recognize when they must refer an individual displaying certain signs and symptoms to other members of the health care team, and how to spot critical red flags as they arise.

Just as there is no reason to believe that a qualified physical therapist cannot be adequately trained to recognize red flags and refer to the relevant providers, there is no reason to believe they will suddenly want to become patients' sole, independent providers, for every condition, in every instance, in all settings. The same is true of nurses.

A truly solo health care practice is actually a canard, particularly as medicine gets more and more complicated. It is virtually impossible to go without input from the histopathologist, for example, to whom the clinician sends their patients' tissue samples for further analysis, or from the radiologist, who ultimately reviews every case that is sent to their service for

MRI, CT or radiograph. Could a surgeon successfully operate without an anesthetist to administer the appropriate anesthesia, or a surgical technologist to prepare the operating theatre? Could a cardiothoracic surgeon reasonably perform a cardiac transplant surgery without a qualified cardiovascular perfusionist to run the bypass machine? Could a general medicine practitioner run a clinic without an infectious disease specialist to turn to with his or her questions, should a particularly complicated infectious disease case arise, for which they are ill-suited to care for alone? Health care is and has always been a team effort. Nothing is done in total solitude, carte blanche. This will never change, and any other imaginable system of healthcare delivery is unsustainable in today's economy. It would be foolish and shortsighted to think that allowing nurse practitioners the freedom to practice with more autonomy what they were educated and trained to do, and which they irrefutably do very well, will upset the current cooperative interdependence that has become the norm in U.S. health care.

To believe that an isolated medical practice could exist appears similar to holding the belief that one could live without the help of anybody else. In reality, we all need our local garbage person, our farmer, our grocer, our mail delivery person and everyone in between to get by successfully. And, realistically, the vast majority of medical practices that employ nurse practitioners, even in the twenty four or so states that do not offer nurses independent practice rights, do not require that physicians tediously scour through the nurses' charts to be sure they haven't made egregious errors, merely that they sign them. But, assuming the seemingly irrational fears of many of the physicians' antagonistic to the idea of the autonomous nurse practitioner should ever see the light of day, what exactly is a signed piece of paper supposed to prevent, if what's on the paper has never been reviewed in the proper sense of the term? Who, or what, exactly is this antiquated system actually protecting, other than perhaps an acknowledgement of superiority?

Competition vs. Collaboration

As was mentioned previously, the dispute here appears to stem predominantly from a feeling that nurse practitioners are stepping on the toes of the physician, who, for various reasons, has had to endure a long and arduous road in order to be able to call himself "the Doctor" and practice medicine at the level they have become accustomed. That said, this aggression seems to be displaced. It is indicative of a turf war, not a legitimate, professional dispute over discrepancies that can be demonstrated concretely by any scientific evidence. If it was, this war would be waged less with heated emotion and legislative battles, and more with data.

Is it possible that the many physicians who are openly angry about autonomous nurse practitioners are merely projecting a form of internal jealousy, as they were forced to endure the painstaking process and crushing debt of medical school, residency, and possibly a fellowship, all for what they may perceive to be "nothing?" Is it possible that some of these providers feel as though, had they known about the so-called "easier" path to practice - which many of them perceive the nursing route to be - they might have decided to travel that path, instead? If so, isn't it plausible that this may be more about themselves and their own discomfort with their decisions, given the state of medical training and health care today, than with nurse practitioners and their ability to provide competent care? Considering the overwhelming data available at present regarding the efficacy and safety of the advanced practice nurse, especially in primary care,[5] it seems doubtful that this debate is really about patient safety, even if that may have been the guise most people have long stood behind when asserting the proposed dichotomies in training between the medical and nursing professions as reason to limit the scope of expanded nursing practice. Unfortunately for the proponents of this stance, the totality of the evidence simply does not favor that position.[5-7]

Whatever the reason, unless or until there is any substantial evidence to suggest that nurse practitioners cannot perform their duties in a high-quality manner, this unfortunate debate, which moves our attention away from patient care and places it onto personal and professional agendas, should be stopped entirely. There is no evidence to suggest that nurse practitioners provide care that is of lower quality than their physician counterparts, and, indeed, there is a significant amount of data that suggests exactly the opposite. See: Horrocks, et al. (2002).[5-7]

Please, do not misunderstand; the implication is not that both professionals are equivalent. Neither could a physician, trained under the medical model of care, hope to perform identically as a nurse practitioner, can the advanced practice nurse expect the opposite to hold true. The suggestion here is merely that the data that would indict the nurse practitioner as being a hazard to patient safety and public health does not exist, and, as such, it is the duty of health care professionals to recognize and appreciate it. It is time we move on and work together to make one another, and each of the health professions better. This should not mean oversight, written protocols and restrictive collaborative agreements, or limitations to anyone's practice, per se. It means being mature enough to recognize that there are instances where physician involvement may be necessary, and, conversely, instances where it should suffice to have a nurse provide autonomous care for certain persons or populations. Let us stop battling back and forth for reasons which run counter to all available evidence, and to the underlying goal of both professions, which is ultimately to keep people happy and healthy.

Identity Crises and Perceived Superiority

It could be argued that one contributing factor to the problem is that a significant number of nurse practitioners try to distance themselves from what they call "regular nurses" - e.g. the traditional, bedside nurse - by claiming that, while a so-called regular RN provides a basic level of nursing-oriented care, they are actually practicing some derivation of medicine. Perhaps this is one understandable reason why so many medical doctors may feel angry or slighted, regarding the scope of practice now accessed and accessible by these nurses. In fact, these professionals do not provide medical care, they are actually trained to utilize some of the tools of medicine to provide advanced nursing care. This is an important distinction. If they were a medical provider, they would have gone to medical or physician assistant school, and been trained under the medical model of care delivery. Rather, they became nurses, and were trained under the nursing model of care, and are thus advanced practice nurses, not medical practitioners - hence the title, *nurse* practitioner. The most important aspect of that title is of course the nurse part, not the advanced practice part. That one possesses the capability to prescribe medications, or diagnose and treat illness, does not change the fact that they ultimately operate from a different philosophical paradigm, or at least were trained to do so.

Regarding the comment made on medical versus nursing practice, the astute reader may contend that a nurse who prescribes medications and manages common diseases is practicing medicine, and that one cannot claim that, simply because their prior training reflects a different paradigm, they are really practicing advanced nursing instead. Although the initial judgement seems to make sense at first glance, I would implore them to consider this further. What, pray tell, is the difference between medicine and nursing, in practice, if not for distinctions in philosophical vantage points? A nurse providing medical care from their perspective as a nurse is as much practicing nursing as a physician carrying out a nursing task in a manner traditionally accomplished by a nurse would still be practicing medicine. For example, let us accept that the average medical doctor can competently insert an intravenous catheter for a blood draw. Since this task is typically completed by an RN, is the physician suddenly practicing nursing by doing it themselves? I suspect the immediate response from many readers would be to say no, given that their training was in medicine. Why, then, does this suddenly change when it is a nurse whose role has expanded? Has it to do with the idea that they are not merely taking on a different role, but a more difficult one, because medicine is inherently more intellectually challenging than nursing? Perhaps it has something to do with the perception that to insert a catheter, as a nurse, is less cerebral than to do so as a physician. Clearly, this is a gross oversimplification of a far more nuanced issue, and the intention is not to downplay it for effect, but to consider the possibility that the underlying perceptions conditioned by our social and cultural views of physicians and nurses may be the driving factors motivating some of these concerns.[8]

This problem of self-aggrandizement and the apparent need to feel superior over other persons in the workplace is rampant in the United States, and is in no way unique to nursing. In fact, it permeates every aspect of health care, from the surgeon who looks down on the general practitioner and views them as less valuable, to the department technician who looks down on the janitorial staff and views them as less valuable. Everyone likes to feel special in their own way, to generate a kind of external validation that makes what they do feel worth it, perhaps reflective of a kind of unexamined existential angst. If this means putting others down so that they may pick themselves up, so be it. But is this really who we want to be, and can we do nothing to curb this kind of petty behavior?

Appeal to Substandard Training

Many people seem to perceive the different physicians as all being rather the same, as in they are all "doctors;" that whatever delineations exist in their practices are minor. However, should you take a moment to speak with a specialist in gastroenterology for any length of time, for example, there is a good chance they may eventually explain how poor of a job the "regular internist" does at diagnosing gastric disorders as compared to the GI fellow. The same goes for the cardiologist, who may suggest that the primary care doctor could never comprehend the cardiovascular system to the same degree they can, because their training is too general. Or the radiologists, who seem to contend that no other physicians truly read radiographs and other imaging studies, like they do. Whether these assertions follow or not is beside the point, but, it must be asked: if this were true, would it mean we should stop allowing the non-specialist physicians to care for patients with the same medical conditions, or interpret the same diagnostic imaging studies, because providers exist with more extensive knowledge in those areas of medicine? Although one does not generally see this argument posited as a limitation to the practice of general medicine physicians, it is often leveled at nurse practitioners and other nurse specialists working in expanded roles. That physician providers exist is not sufficient reason to prohibit the nurse practitioner from performing those tasks which are within their scope of practice and for which they were trained to do, merely because they were educated differently. For this stance to be held, a well-reasoned and evidence-based argument that, as compared to physicians, nurses provide inadequate patient care in the relevant contexts, ought to accompany it. Again, there is no evidence for this purported phenomenon in the primary literature.

If the argument against nurse practitioners is about physicians having received better training - ignoring the nondescript nature of that sentiment - then why stop at schooling? Why not take this line of logic even further and suggest, for example, that because med-peds physicians get a greater depth and breadth of internal medicine training for both adults and children that family physicians ought not practice internal medicine and pediatrics anymore? Or that because an ophthalmologist is better trained at treating eye pathology than a geriatrician, that geriatricians may no longer utilize their knowledge of ocular disease to treat glaucoma, but must instead refer to a specialist? Or that because clinical immunologists are the resident experts in the study of asthma and allergy, the primary care physician should be barred from treating those conditions in the outpatient setting, without referring to an allergy clinic? Needless to say, this would be viewed as an outrageous and absurd idea, and yet those who would have you believe that nurse practitioners should not be allowed to practice to the full extent of their license fall back on the same belief, that because physicians may have more in-depth training in human disease in medical school, the nurse ought not treat the same conditions.

As an aside, the above notion speaks to the Naturalistic fallacy, or the ought-is problem. By which I mean, just because it *ought* to be the case that physicians are better trained providers than nurses does not mean that it *is* the case that they are superior providers. The same goes for the various specialist physicians. Just because a full-fledged cardiothoracic surgeon ought to better understand the anatomy and physiology of the heart than a third year medical student does not mean that this is the case, in reality. Further examples could be carried on, ad nauseam.

One legitimate concern leveled at advanced practice nurses describes the hypothetical practitioner, who, perhaps due to their own feelings of self-importance, chooses not to refer their more complicated cases out to more experienced providers, when they are out of their depth. Frankly, physicians must also learn to acknowledge when they are out of their depth in precisely the same way, and be willing to refer to other members of the health care team when it would most benefit their patient. As health care providers, it is the duty of both physicians and nurses alike to check their egos at the door. But, to the multitude of physicians who are openly and vocally concerned that this will become a bigger problem with respect to nurses providing more advanced care, there does not seem to be any compelling reason to believe that nurses are not already recognizing their limitations and referring appropriately. In fact, there is some conflicting data to suggest that primary care nurses refer more frequently than their physician counterparts,[9-10] which would seem to imply a relative lack of the egoism of concern, here.

The Ideology of the Nurse Practitioner as a Midlevel

It has become common to refer to nurse practitioners as *midlevel providers*, or *physician extenders*. The insinuation, by referring to an advanced practice nurse as a midlevel provider, is not only offensive in connotation, but implies that anyone lower on the practitioner totem pole somehow provides substandard care, which gets poorer and poorer, as one trends downward. By this logic, physicians provide top-tier patient care, nurse practitioners and physician assistants sub-optimal care, and registered nurses mediocre care.

This particular conception is rather asinine. Healthcare is not a totem pole, or a pyramid, with the physician sitting at the top, like the ship's captain; a god-like pinnacle of expertise and professionalism, and all other practitioners falling in line beneath Him. The truth looks more like an interprofessional spider chart, with the patient at the center, and everyone else working together to improve the life of that person, their family and the community. In an ideal world, the individual philosophies of all hospital personnel would change to reflect this reality, in order to make for a more efficient and effective approach to health care delivery for everyone.

It is this author's belief that the term midlevel provider arose out of an inappropriate conflation between nurse practitioners and certified physician assistants (PA-C). Briefly, without getting into a detailed history comparing and contrasting the two professions, the physician assistant began as exactly that described above, an extension of the physician - in the U.S. Military - in order to lighten his workload and assist with simpler cases, so the doctor might focus his attention on the more complex ones. Ignoring the fact that the role of the physician assistant has since expanded far beyond that, and despite the slow, progressive move toward the adoption of the more liberal title, physician *associate*, the physician assistant still functions, and will always function, as an extension of the physician; hence the implication in the job title. The problem here is that people often conflate the types of work performed by physician assistants and nurse practitioners, because they are so similar - even though it is sometimes forgotten that, with particular regard for primary care, neither are much different from the role of the physician. Thus, they are viewed as the same, and since the medical establishment views the physician assistant as subservient to the physician (rather than an equal extension, on par with the medical doctor, but with a different scope), they also view the nurse practitioner as subservient. e.g. If the NP and the PA have the same role, these professionals must be the same, and since the level of care provided by the PA is (in their minds) lesser than the physician, it must be fair to categorize them both as midlevel providers, since physicians have long been considered advanced or expert providers. The multiple flaws in this line of reasoning should be quite transparent.

Philosophical Differences: Biomedical vs. Biopsychosocial

It would be remiss of me to ignore the differences in academic training that do currently exist between nursing and medicine. However, although one must acknowledge that there is an information gap in the pre-clinical training period between these two fields of study, this is by no means an insurmountable disparity; and it is being dealt with in other ways, as the demand for a higher level of nursing education, both in academia and in clinical practice, continues to grow. I do not wish to delve too deeply into the intricacies of this particular topic, although it is an interesting and important consideration for future papers. Instead, I should like to touch briefly on the differences in the philosophy of care that distinguishes nursing from medicine.

While medicine traditionally focuses on the disease state, or "the disease a person has," nursing focuses largely on the healing of the whole person; "a person who has a disease." Pragmatically-speaking, both approaches amount to roughly the same thing: the eradication of disease, so the patient may return to their life a healthier human being. Philosophically, the implications are more nuanced, with nursing modalities often favoring a value-laden system of care sometimes referred to as the biopsychosocial model, initially postulated by the late American Psychiatrist, Dr. George Engel.[11]

Where modern medicine is concerned, Engel's biopsychosocial model - perhaps better termed *perspective* or *hypothesis*[12] - has long been usurped by the more traditional biomedical model of care, wherein the primary focus is to develop an intricate understanding of pathology, often at the exclusion of other psychological, social, politico-economic, or ethical factors that may play an important role. Nursing, on the other hand, has kept the biopsychosocial model alive, and it seems to be a fundamental driver of the underlying philosophy of the profession.

More often than not, it seems that the various branches of medicine choose to focus on the eradication of disease to sustain life, irrespective of any other factor. In other words, do whatever is necessary to keep the cells and tissues functioning for as long as possible, in every attempt to stave off death. Thus, one might go so far as to claim that while medicine's focus is to increase the *lifespan* of an organism, nursing's focus is to promote a person's *healthspan* - despite an urgent need to better and more comprehensively understand this latter term[13]; suggesting that the disease process is secondary to the individual who has befallen it.

Perhaps overly simplistic, those in medicine tend to focus primarily on curing disease, whereas the focus of nursing is on healing the individual and restoring a person's capacity to function. The physician is trained to diagnose and treat specific pathologies. Should they be successful in accomplishing this often perilous feat, their job is largely done. In contrast, nurses are trained to view the individual as a whole, taking into account their environmental well-being, their family dynamics, the biological realities of their disease and the patient's own phenomenological experience of that reality, which is why nursing is widely considered to be more holistic than medicine.[14-16] The ultimate goal of the physician is to cure disease. The goal of the nurse is to maximize patient outcomes by working to increase self-efficacy and optimize self-actualization, of which having an understanding of the disease process and treatment planning is only one aspect. Whereas medicine is intrinsically disease-centered, nursing is person-centered. This is not to insinuate that there are not physicians who practice in a holistic, patient-centered manner. This is merely meant to suggest that, from the standpoint of their education and training, physicians are not typically exposed to the same theoretical principles that nurses are.[17] The important thing to acknowledge here, is that, even though the clinical roles of physicians and nurse practitioners may overlap at times, and are similar in some familiar ways, there are important distinctions between the ways they are taught to think about patient care.

It must be reiterated that the above statements are not aimed at all (or indeed any) physicians, as individual providers. (Neither, is it meant to demean or otherwise diminish the unique complexity of medical science, which can also be challenging to define and nail down in its own concrete ontology.) It is clear that there are in fact many individual physicians who practice in a similar fashion, and they are to be commended. But the establishment to which they are attached and from which they were trained does not necessarily endorse this philosophical approach to patient care as readily as the nursing profession does.[18]

These distinctions, while important in their own right, are just that; philosophical. Again, I think it is important to inquire as to: what is the difference between nursing and medicine, if not for the philosophies that underpin them? Where would one drawn the line between "while X is a nursing task, Y is a medical task," if there were not these value-laden boundaries we subjectively and somewhat arbitrarily assign, by virtue of their philosophical implications and our own in-grouping ideals?

Regression to the Mean

Some medical schools are beginning to realize the importance of treating the whole person, and not just their symptoms or systemic illnesses, and that, on the other side of their diagnoses and treatment plans lies a real person, with feelings and experiences, who exists in a lively and adaptive social environment, all of which is impacted by their interventions. Hence, from 2015 on, the Medical College Admissions Test (MCAT) has been changed accordingly to incorporate more psychology, behavioral health, and human growth and development, in lieu of additional molecular biology and physics,[19] and many pre-medical requirements are changing, in long overdue response to an evolving health care climate.[20-21]

Although certain physician advocacy groups like to boast that their arduous, four year medical education properly prepares physicians to safely care for people and their families, [22] there are at least three programs that confer the M.D. degree to motivated medical students who know they are interested in pursuing primary care in three years of abbreviated study.[23-25] As of yet, there are no exceptional data examining the effects of these novel programs on patient health and safety, but it is interesting that the time investment and length of training for these programs - which one would like to assume produces equally qualified medical graduates - is slowly starting to resemble the average three-year masters of nursing science degree that confers the entry-level nurse practitioner certification. Could it be that primary care is a unique specialty unto itself that requires a specific body of knowledge and skills, which need not necessarily take four years of diverse medical education and a three year residency in order to practice safely and effectively? The American Academy of Family Physicians (AAFP), for instance, reproachfully argues against the autonomous nurse practitioner, because family physicians typically accumulate an average of 20,000 hours of hands-on clinical practice during their residencies, while the average nurse practitioner gets "just 1,000 hours" during their master's program.[22] Irrespective of the fact that these smear campaigns intentionally omit the many years of clinical experience most nurses have gained prior to nurse practitioner school, isn't it also possible that a primary care provider may not necessarily require so many supervised clinical hours to practice competently? The data in favor of nurse practitioners, which are plentiful, would seem to support this assertion.

Given these progressivist changes, both to the MCAT and to pre- and post-graduate medical education, and that the graduate education of nurses is steadily improving, it appears there is a kind of regression to the mean happening. Considering this as a possibility, it is tempting to ask whether this debate is even worth having anymore.

The Best and Brightest

It is often stated that the "best and brightest" go to medical school, while those who can't hack the MCAT or the intense seven-to-ten year commitment that follows it go into nursing, instead. Although there is no objective evidence to speak to this phenomenon, let us briefly examine this judgmental, intrinsically-sexist concept, so as to move beyond it and broach a mutual understanding.

Direct-entry masters degree (and more recently doctoral degree) programs in nursing are now available at many U.S. universities, whereby the degree is conferred, after two-four years (or approximately 77-130 credits) of advanced training in a specialized area of nursing practice, beyond the baccalaureate level. Prior to entry into these competitive programs, all of the matriculants must meet a specified set of prerequisite guidelines, as well as having already achieved a bachelors degree in a field other than nursing. Although the minimum grade point average requirement for matriculation is a 3.0, and although the personnel who review each case take more into consideration than just a prospective student's academic background, it is a rare event that the accepted individuals have earned less than a 3.4 cumulative GPA.[26]

Despite the malicious and unfounded assumption that medical students are generally smarter than nursing students, out of the 177 schools across the United States that currently offer the M.D. or D.O. degrees, 29% have an average incoming GPA between 2.7 and 3.7.[27] Out of the 35 D.O. schools in the United States, 46% have an average incoming GPA of less than 3.4.[27]

After seeing these figures, some might scoff and suggest this is not a fair comparison, because medical students must first take and do well on the MCAT, prior to acceptance into medical school, and then take and pass the USMLE Steps 1, 2 and 3, before becoming attending physicians. Setting aside the important fact that nursing and medicine, although they overlap in some significant ways, are different fields of study, both in theory and in practice, and ought to be governed independently of one another, nurses have to pass rigorous standardized examinations in order to prove themselves capable of practice, as well. (Whether they are "as rigorous," aside from being an untestable, unscientific question, is another matter altogether.)

Keeping with our example, a direct-entry masters degree student hopeful, before getting accepted into the nursing program, must take and do well on the Graduate Record Examination (GRE), to prove their capacity to study at the graduate school level. Then, typically before the start of their second year, they must take and pass the NCLEX-RN examination for registered nurses. Once they have graduated from the program, and go on to become certified in their specialty, they must take and pass the AANP or ANCC board examinations in their respective areas of expertise. They then have a five year period between their first certification and when they must re-certify, which requires not only being able to pass the exam again, but also accumulating a certain number of continuing education units in order to be eligible to retake the test.

Frankly, as this author finds these points trivial and meaningless without specific context, it would be interesting to know how many licensed physicians could pass the USMLE step 1, ten years out of medical school, with the same grade they achieved the first time around. It is a well-described psychological phenomenon that people tend to retain and best recall the information they use repeatedly, whereas memories that have not been accessed regularly tend to decay continuously with the passage of time.[28] Perhaps this is one of the many possible reasons the data surrounding standard medical care versus advanced nursing care appear indistinguishable, regardless of the outcome measure in question.[7] Again, I should like to point to regression to the mean as a potential culprit.

Is it really important for a medical practitioner to know, offhand, that the intravenous catheter they are inserting into a patient's arm is composed of polytetrafluoroethylene? How clinically relevant is ones prior knowledge of buoyant forces or intricate organocatalysis to a patient who comes into the clinic with a diffuse, erythematous rash? I am not questioning the underlying pertinence of these scientific concepts to physiology, nor am I suggesting that their connections to clinical medicine cannot be made, on some level.

I am questioning, as I think we ought to, the direct relevance of ones familiarity with these bits of information to specific cases, and whether knowing them has any measurable impact on patient outcomes, in clinical practice.

However difficult it may be for some to accept, the truth is that the so-called "best and brightest" flood both occupations, and have highly personal and individual reasons for choosing careers in either medicine or nursing, which may say absolutely nothing about their IQs. The fact of the matter is, as we all know, there are wonderful nurses and wonderful physicians, as well, unfortunately, as poor nurses and poor physicians. It all boils down to the person who holds the title, not the title itself. To insinuate that nursing is a career for those who were not bright enough to succeed in medicine is not only untrue, it is demeaning.

Intellect is Person-Dependent, Not Degree-Dependent

Especially in the United States, it seems to be a universally held belief that the more advanced someone's academic background, the more intelligent they are.

An educational program, however important in the training of a competent individual in any field of study, is insufficient, by itself, to confer proficiency or expertise in a given area, including human health. There must first be a person with adequate mental faculties with which to organize, synthesize and assimilate the requisite information to memory, and then use it consistently, over a long period of time, to maintain it. It would be an unfair generalization to suggest that the physician is inherently more knowledgeable on the subject of medicine, as a whole, than persons in other health professions, simply because they attended medical school.

Arduous though traditional medical training may be, the most important and often overlooked concept here is that there is always a human being to whose name the accolade M.D. is attached. If one momentarily ignores the sheet of paper certifying this person's noble achievement, one is forced to recognize that, ultimately, the intellect and aptitude of this individual and their ability to perform the functions of a medical provider rest solely on their mental faculties. It is not predicated, as is so often assumed, on which college degree they have received, from what institution.

The arguments here, and all those to follow, are not aimed at discrediting or discriminating against one healthcare professional or another, or suggesting that one training style over another is somehow better. It is merely being posited that it first takes a conscious and intelligent person to provide medical care, and that, without this thinking, feeling, relating human being, the alphabet soup that pays homage to a title after their name is surely meaningless.

What Factors Govern Expertise?

Let us briefly examine a member of the interdisciplinary health care team, who is somewhat removed from and therefore relatively neutral to nursing and medicine; namely, the Clinical Laboratory Scientist.

Clinical laboratory scientists are licensed health care professionals and experts in the laboratory diagnosis of disease. It has been said that something approximating 80% of the diseases that healthcare practitioners diagnose would be impossible without the help of a qualified laboratory scientist.[29] Their training is typically limited to a baccalaureate degree in a biological science, and they take an exorbitant number of complex, post-graduate courses in histology, immunobiology, clinical chemistry, pathophysiology, and more. Despite the fact that a vast majority of these professionals do not hold advanced degrees, they are widely considered the autonomous experts in laboratory diagnosis.

The question being wrung from this information is whether one would be willing to suggest that a physician is inherently more qualified to provide insights into the laboratory results of a sick patient than the clinical laboratory scientist, simply in virtue of his or her being a physician? Considering the laboratory scientist performs tasks highly specific to this area of medicine, on a daily basis, and has an intimate understanding of the complicated mechanisms underpinning the diseases they help to diagnose, it is difficult to imagine many physicians who would lay claim to possessing more knowledge on such topics, merely by having ascertained a medical degree.

Another example that serves the present argument is the paramedic, who has practical, hands-on experience, on a daily basis, resuscitating people with continuously refined life support techniques. It is difficult to imagine a dermatologist knowing more about emergency medical management than a paramedic, with 1/10th the level of pre-clinical education, simply because it is not information they study and apply on a daily basis. Equally as absurd, of course, would be the assumption that a paramedic could gestalt recognize a malignant melanoma, like a dermatologist could. Or, for that matter, that a medical intensivist could do the same. Their areas of specialization, and thus their clinical expertise are quite different.

Imagine a family physician, in a busy, suburban clinic, who has been in practice for fifteen years, and hasn't sewn up a skin laceration since their residency. Would it be fair to say that, because they can write the letters M.D. after their name, they are better prepared than a surgical physician assistant to suture a complex laceration? What about a pediatrician who works with a pediatric nurse practitioner, who, for the last decade, has maintained a specialized focus on the management of kids with congenital cardiac defects. Does this nurse's physician colleague know more about congenital heart abnormalities, intrinsically, than she, simply because they are a physician? Will a physician in the emergency department, trained primarily as a resuscitationist, recognize and be able to differentiate between early-stage diabetic retinopathy and diffuse unilateral subacute neuroretinitis, as readily as their ophthalmology colleagues?

Consider that every newly-minted family physician, fresh out of residency, has had some level of neurosurgical experience, at some point in their medical training. It seems reasonable to ask whether this information is useful, in the context of primary care, or if we are merely perpetuating an archaic, antiquated tradition for its own sake?

a.) The general practitioner will almost assuredly never utilize their neurosurgical skills, again, throughout the duration of their careers - assuming they collected any of these "skills" to begin with.

b.) One may not need formal neurosurgical training to recognize critical red flags and refer neuro- patients for immediate consults with the appropriate providers.

c.) Even if the need to call on this information should ever arise for some reason, it is unreasonable to suspect that a sufficient amount of neurosurgery knowledge would be remembered to competently perform the necessary procedure. Surgery is a rapidly changing field of medicine, and the techniques used in 1978 are likely to be dramatically different, and far less safe and effective, than those taught in 2015.

Does a physician inherently know more clinical pharmacology than the practicing clinical pharmacist? Are they automatically more proficient at drawing blood than the phlebotomist, with 2,000 hours of experience per annum doing so, or at identifying a partial medial meniscus tear, as compared to a licensed physical therapist? Will a pediatric endocrinologist more quickly recognize a gradually decompensating pulmonary patient compared to the respiratory therapist of thirty years?

Physicians are imperative to the quality of patient care, and integral to the health care system, and no one is denying that, but it must be remembered that they too are only human and are trained as specialists for a reason. No single individual can possibly know everything, particularly in a field as complicated as medicine. Ascertaining the M.D. degree does not miraculously confer superhuman faculties.

Is there provider oversight in the behavioral health sciences, where a psychiatrist oversees the practice of so-called "midlevel" practitioners? Do psychiatrists and psychotherapists battle over who does the job better, as physicians and nurse practitioners do, in primary care? To assume that mental health providers are not subject to the same level of professional responsibility as a medical provider is narrow-minded thinking, and the former is an area dominated by the masters level clinician, not the physician. Despite this, there appears to be far more amicable tendencies between the mental health specialists. Could the same feat be accomplished in clinical medicine?

Whatever ones area of clinical expertise, most of a clinician's learning is not done in the classroom, but on the job. In fact, it is quite common for attending physicians to claim that they did not really become a physician until somewhere in their residency. The hands on, practical application of information is where the true assimilation of a great deal of a clinician's knowledge takes place. For instance, would it be wise to blindly trust the opinion of a green PGY-2 internist in the ICU, over that of an RN with fifteen years of high-acuity, critical care experience under their belt? In fact, what is the difference, really, between the physician and the nurse of this caliber, if we ignore that much of the legal responsibility is currently shouldered by the physician? Medically, it seems that both parties would likely have a similar practical knowledge base, due to their respective levels of experience, not their previous collegiate coursework. It is easy to imagine that a majority of this information may have been quickly forgotten, shortly after graduation, anyway. As they say, ones education starts when school ends. (Or, perhaps better stated, school is a necessary but insufficient component of ones education.)

Perhaps the most frustrating of many things people often fail to take into account in this discussion is the apparent inability of physician groups to recognize just how much clinical experience nurses have, and that spending ten years as a board certified family nurse practitioner, is, in some ways, akin to having completed a family medicine residency of their own, similar in scope, but with different philosophical and practical implications. An often overlooked reality, for those who would wish to deny nurse practitioners more autonomy and the right to practice to the full extent of their license, is that, while a physician's specialty training does not begin until the start of their residency program, a nurse practitioner, from the day they enter the classroom, has already dedicated themselves to a particular nursing specialty.

A Futile Dispute Over the Clinical Doctorate

In order to have a meaningful discussion on the topic of who gets to call himself *doctor*, and what factors distinguish a medical school graduate from a nursing school graduate, we must first define our terms, and then appropriately differentiate one plan of study from the other.

From an etymological perspective, the word doctor, from its latin derivation, *docere*, actually means *teacher*. It is for this reason that when a person is awarded a Ph.D. degree from an accredited university, they are thereafter referred to as a doctor. It is not that they have become a clinician, and can make diagnoses on other human beings, per se, but that they have completed a level of education such that they may be considered an expert, a teacher. In no way do physicians have a monopoly over this term.

A doctoral degree is awarded when a person completes a specific set of graduate-level courses and, usually, defends some kind of a thesis or dissertation, or otherwise completes a scholarly project, and is then, upon completion of said requirements, awarded a doctorate in that area of study. Thus, they are thereafter able to refer to themselves, and rightly so by this standard, as *doctor*. If having achieved a doctorate is sufficient for most other professionals to call themselves doctor, and the etymological definition of the term means teacher, why is it that physicians claim ownership to the title, or have a problem with graduates of the doctor of nursing practice (D.N.P.) degree program being called doctor?

From a historical standpoint, doctors who have fulfilled clinical roles in healthcare have mostly been physicians. It makes sense, therefore, that today's physicians might reject or refuse to accept another practitioner with so much practical overlap as the nurse practitioner from being appointed a clinical doctorate, and thus invading their territory. After all, a similar battle raged on for many years, after the osteopathic (D.O.) movement came along and did largely the same thing. Considering this, one might posit that the real concern stems from the same beliefs generated by the faulty generalizations previously mentioned in this paper. (Interestingly, a vital difference between what happened with the osteopathic movement and what is currently happening with the nursing movement is that nurse practitioners are not trying to become physicians, whereas osteopaths were and did.)

With the comparison of "M.D. *versus* D.N.P.," we already have a conflation happening. This is incorrect thinking, from the start, as both degrees set out to educate trainees in substantially different ways. If one examines the curriculum of the D.N.P. degree in any detail, they may notice that it does not appear to include any more advanced courses in clinical medicine, as a physician advocate group might have it, which seems to be the primary motive for physicians to denounce the legitimacy of the degree. There is a reason for this, however: the educational models of medical school and nursing school are intentionally different; yet again, recall that they are different professions. Their leadership roles and clinical functions are different, and, therefore, their educational paradigms reflect this difference. At present, there is no objective evidence that a masters level nurse practitioner should require any more advanced biomedical courses, pertinent to their specialty, than they have already taken, in order to practice safely and effectively. However, there is an increasing need for these advanced practice nurses to be able to competently analyze nursing research and translate it into clinical practice. Considering that a nurse practitioner is a specialty provider, right out of graduate school, they ought to be held to the same standard as other specialists, whether medical or ancillary, who must keep up with the ever-expanding knowledge base from which they are expected to practice.

The aim of the doctor of nursing practice is to prime advanced practice nurses with the tools necessary to lead healthcare teams, help patients navigate the convoluted healthcare system, mentor and educate budding nurses, and, perhaps most importantly of all, to keep up with and translate population-specific nursing research into clinical practices. Translational research and the implementation of these data is arguably one of the strongest features of the D.N.P. program. Where the Ph.D. in nursing science prepares the nurse researcher to conduct these sorts of studies, and generate original data, the DNP prepares the advanced practice nurse and clinical nurse leader to take these data and translate them to the bedside, improving and contributing to patient outcomes, through evidence-based practice.

Many people would assert that the problem is physicians are outraged that a provider with less training than them is being allowed to practice in a similar capacity. I would contend that, although there may be some truth to that, other factors should be considered as well - e.g. Not just ones level of education, but their specificity of their training, as well. For instance, there are family physicians who argue that obstetrician-gynecologists, who can and often do act as primary care providers for women, should not be allowed to function in this role, given that they are not legitimate primary care providers.[30] However, an Ob/Gyn physician has had the same four-year undergraduate medical education as the family physician, and then a four-year residency in obstetrics and gynecology, possibly followed by a one to three year fellowship in a variety of sub-specialty areas. Arguably then, the attending Ob/Gyn has likely had *more* training in women's health, both reproductive and non-reproductive, than the the typical, outpatient general practitioner; even though the argument is that the former's training is less specific to outpatient primary care medicine. Because the family physician does not view the "role" of the Ob/Gyn to be that of general practitioner, they feel their Ob/Gyn colleagues ought not provide such general care to their patients, as it might do them "a disservice."[30]

Did these physicians not get the exact same medical education? Clearly, there is more at play here than physicians merely having accumulated more training hours than nurses, or having achieved a higher level of education. And, if it were merely about having a wealth of experience in a particular clinical setting, as the aforementioned argument might imply, surely the nurse practitioner has had that part covered all along. So, what exactly is the real concern, here?

It seems physicians are trying to reflect on the DNP in light of the medical model of care, to which they are so strongly accustomed and conditioned to believe is the only sensible model to follow. Whereas a doctor of medicine is taught to translate *medical* research to the bedside, a doctor of nursing practice is taught to translate *nursing* research to the bedside; which may or may not include similar kinds of trials - as biomedical scientists and nurse scientists tend to work together on various projects. But, as they are not well-versed in this area of health science, these physicians do as most people do, when they do not understand something; reject it.

The other issue to consider is the implicit assumption from many professionals that the DNP is correlated specifically with nurse practitioners, but one need not be an advanced practice registered nurse to become a DNP. There are avenues for registered nurses and clinical nurse leaders to advance their careers by ascertaining the doctorate degree. Again, just because various nursing organizations wish the D.N.P. degree to be the entry-level degree to advanced clinical practice does not necessitate that that practice be of the same kind provided by nurse practitioners. (Indeed, the pathways to DNP include: registered nurses, clinical nurse leaders, clinical nurse specialists, certified nurse midwives, certified registered nurse anesthetists *and* nurse practitioners.)

The aim of the D.N.P. is to funnel nurses into leadership positions and increase the competency of nurses in providing unparalleled *nursing* care, whether clinically advanced or not, and translating *nursing* research to the patients' bedside, whether diagnostic or not. To reiterate: The DNP is about advanced nursing practice, not advanced nurse practitioner practice. The degree was not designed to compete with medical graduates. The medical model of care and medical doctors were not even factored into its development, other than as one of many examples of various other professionals who happen to hold doctorate degrees in the clinic.

Meet Doctor Nurse

One of the most widely cited reasons for rejecting the DNP seems to be that if there are two doctors in the clinical setting, patients will get confused as to who is the "real doctor" is. Or, rather, that they will not know how to properly differentiate between the advanced practice nurse and the physician.

The unfortunate belief, implicit in this argument, presupposes that the American people are not intelligent enough to distinguish between two distinct healthcare professionals, who happen to hold different doctoral degrees. Perhaps it is true that, every so often, an individual may be confused by the difference - and, naturally, the lay public should not be expected to know precisely what the DNP is, or how it explicitly differs from the MD - but it is unreasonable to suppose that such an individual is incapable of asking for the physician, should they be uncomfortable with the care provided by a nurse, or vice versa. Secondly, in this technologically advanced age, every one of us is lucky enough to have access to the same information, online. Should they be so motivated as to find out for themselves just what these differences in training and practice are, they have access to that information, at any time, including at their bedside from their cell phones. It is their own prerogative, should they choose to investigate further, and be an advocate in their own care. But, it is unfair and insulting to suspect that the average American adult could not adequately differentiate an advanced practice nurse from a physician, when he or she enters the room and says, "Hello, my name is Dr. X, I'll be your nurse practitioner," and is wearing a name tag that reads: *Dr. X, nurse practitioner* on it. Most patients can see the difference quite plainly, for themselves, without our having to dumb it down for them, and the majority of people do not care, so long as they are afforded the appropriate health care in their time of need.

Even still, the typical DNP holder does not seem terribly concerned about their ability to use the title doctor in the clinical setting. This does not appear to be especially high on their list of priorities, right now. As is the case with the masters level nurse practitioner, advanced practice nurses who hold the DNP degree are really only fighting for the ability to practice to the full extent of their license, which they naturally believe is their right - and it would not be any more expanded than the masters-level nurse practitioners' scope. With the striking explosion of primary care needs not being met, and a massive and compounding hole in the ability of physicians to supply the demand for this care, which is only expected to worsen over time, the doctorally-prepared nurse will not only be ready for this important responsibility, they will be well-suited to help bridge this gap.

Just as the nurse practitioner knows he or she is not a physician, and does not wish to be, the DNP knows they are not an MD, and does not wish to be. To think otherwise is to continue to propagate a fallacious image of nurses who are unsatisfied with who they are and the kind of work they do. It just so happens that, due to a growing need for medical providers, some of the work that has historically belonged to one profession, and work that has traditionally been integral to the other, has started to overlap in both.

The second most popular reason for fighting against the DNP seems to be based on the claim that it is merely a reflection of a kind of unnecessary degree inflation that is happening throughout the country, so that universities can drum up tens of thousands of extra tuition dollars per year, and that, in terms of practical usefulness, the degree itself is unhelpful. This belief appears to be due to a lack of understanding as to the type and importance of the information that DNP programs impart on their students. As was already alluded to, the DNP is not about replacing physicians, or stepping in line with the medical model. It is about increasing the leadership potential of the advanced practice nurse, or clinical nurse leader, and facilitating a greater understanding of both medical and nursing care in their respective areas of expertise, and reconciling various aspects of the U.S. healthcare system with the biopsychosocial needs of the people and patients within it.

On some level, there may be a certain amount of degree inflation occurring in the United States, but, if this is true, it is not unique to nursing. Perhaps the reason has more to do with the realization that every area of health science must meet an ever-increasing demand for higher-level knowledge. The following is a list of practice-oriented doctorate degrees currently offered at major U.S. universities:

- Doctor of Medicine (MD)
- Doctor of Osteopathic Medicine (DO)
- Doctor of Dentistry (DMD/DDS)
- Doctor of Podiatric Medicine (DPM)
- Doctor of Optometry (OD)
- Doctor of Education (EdD)
- Doctor of Clinical Psychology (PsyD)

- Doctor of Social Work (DSW)
- Doctor of Marriage & Family Therapy (DMFT)
- Doctor of Health Science (DHS)
- Doctor of Public Health (DrPH)
- Doctor of Occupational Therapy (DOT)
- Doctor of Physical Therapy (DPT)
- Doctor of Clinical Laboratory Science (DCLS)
- Doctor of Clinical Nutrition (DCN)
- Doctor of Chiropractic (DC)

How can someone rationalize jokes at the expense of a nursing professional by making snide comments about "Dr. Nurse," and yet accept that so many other professionals, many of them in fields that directly impact patient care, but none of whom are physicians, have been steadily advancing their knowledge base, in an attempt to increase proficiency and expertise, by awarding doctoral degrees? Why should the doctor of nursing practice be any different?

The Silver Lining

In the end, the most important consideration, much more than any of the other things that have been discussed, is the patient. And not just the quality of care they receive, but that they in fact receive any care at all.

Health care in the United States, as it is currently practiced, is unsustainable and unquestioningly failing millions of people. Preventive care and health maintenance through regular screenings and physical examinations, as well as countless other important medical practices integral to the wellness of every American citizen is dwindling, to the point that *most* people are not being properly taken care of. These roles, particularly in underserved areas, can be filled, successfully, by nurse practitioners, who are already independent providers of high-quality care in the United States and abroad. Luckily for the American public, who are already suffering under the weight of a virtually insurmountable national debt, nurse practitioners also provide demonstrably cost-effective care, as evidenced by a recent systematic review in the British Medical Journal.[31]

Healthcare is a right, not a privilege. There are decades of research in the peer-reviewed literature, despite some methodological limitations, which clearly demonstrate that nurse practitioners provide excellent patient care, in a variety of clinical settings, both collaboratively and autonomously.[5-7] Something must be done, and quickly, to rectify the steadily worsening shortage of qualified providers, as the need for primary care continues to increase at such an astounding rate.[32] Because of their advanced clinical preparation, their holistic practice style, and the sheer size of the nursing profession and its capacity to implement far-reaching changes in the healthcare system, nurses are in a wonderful position to markedly impact this problem in a positive way.[33]

Removing the limitations of the nurse practitioners' ability to practice to the full extent of their license, as one possible strategy in stemming the bleeding that has befallen U.S. primary care, is a good start.[34] It is something, at the very least, that may remove the barrier to care that so many are faced with, around the nation. If we, as scientists and healthcare professionals, could look beyond our own fears and desires, and work together as part of an integrated health care team for the good of the patient, perhaps we could solve this problem after all. It seems reasonable to suggest, given everything discussed at length, above, that the nurse practitioner should be released from the restrictions that currently bind their practice, insofar as it does not correlate sufficiently well with their level of education, or the data regarding their clinical competence. Frankly, it is shameful and impeding the access of millions of Americans to receiving care. It also seems obvious that, for this to happen, we must stop arguing with one another, and shift our focus toward a more utilitarian approach, wherein we work as a cohesive unit, for the good of all patients and the community. We need all hands on deck, especially on the front lines.

Disclosures

None declared.

References

1. "Historical Timeline." *American Association of Nurse Practitioners*. AANP, n.d. Web. 19 June 2015. <http://www.aanp.org/all-about-nps/historical-timeline>.
2. "Nonphysician Practitioners - Relevant Society Position Statements." AMDA, 19 June 2015. Web. <https://www.amda.com/advocacy/Society.cfm?printPage=1&>.
3. "AMA Responds to IOM Report on Future of Nursing." AMA Responds to IOM Report on Future of Nursing. American Medical Association, n.d. Web. 19 June 2015. <http://www.ama-assn.org/ama/pub/news/news/nursing-future-workforce.page>.
4. Deyle, G. D. (2006). Direct access physical therapy and diagnostic responsibility: the risk-to-benefit ratio. *Journal of Orthopaedic & Sports Physical Therapy*, 36(9), 632-634.

5. Laurant, M., Reeves, D., Hermens, R., Braspenning, J., Grol, R., & Sibbald, B. (2005). Substitution of doctors by nurses in primary care. *Cochrane Database Syst Rev*, 2(2).
6. Horrocks, S., Anderson, E., & Salisbury, C. (2002). Systematic review of whether nurse practitioners working in primary care can provide equivalent care to doctors. *BMJ*, 324 (7341), 819-823.
7. Newhouse, R. P., Stanik-Hutt, J., White, K. M., Johantgen, M., Bass, E. B., Zangaro, G., ... & Weiner, J. P. (2011). Advanced practice nurse outcomes 1990-2008: a systematic review. *Nursing Economics*, 29(5), 230.
8. Sweet, S. J., & Norman, I. J. (1995). The nurse-doctor relationship: a selective literature review. *Journal of advanced nursing*, 22(1), 165-170.
9. Liddy, C., Deri Armstrong, C., McKellips, F., & Keely, E. (2015). A comparison of referral patterns to a multispecialty eConsultation service between nurse practitioners and family physicians: The case for eConsult. *Journal of the American Association of Nurse Practitioners*.
10. Mackey, T. A., Cole, F., & Veeser, P. (1999). Nurse practitioner referral patterns in primary care/occupational health care settings. *The Internet Journal of Advanced Nursing Practice*, 2(2).
11. Engel, G. L. (1980). The clinical application of the biopsychosocial model. *Am J Psychiatry*, 137(5), 535-544.
12. McLaren, N. (2009). A critical review of the biopsychosocial model. *Australian and New Zealand Journal of Psychiatry*. Chicago
13. Tatar, M. (2009). Can we develop genetically tractable models to assess healthspan (rather than life span) in animal models?. *The Journals of Gerontology Series A: Biological Sciences and Medical Sciences*, gln067.
14. Woods, S. (1998). Holism in nursing. *In Philosophical Issues in Nursing* (pp. 67-87). Macmillan Education UK.
15. Povlsen, L., & Borup, I. K. (2011). Holism in nursing and health promotion: distinct or related perspectives?–A literature review. *Scandinavian journal of caring sciences*, 25(4), 798-805.
16. Griffin, A. (1992). Holism in nursing: its meaning and value. *British journal of nursing* (Mark Allen Publishing), 2(6), 310-312.
17. Adler, R. H. (2009). Engel's biopsychosocial model is still relevant today. *Journal of psychosomatic research*, 67(6), 607-611.
18. Shaver, J. L. (1985). A biopsychosocial view of human health. An effective approach to nursing care must encompass all factors that act, either singly or in combination, on human health. *Nursing Outlook*, 33(4), 186-191.

19. "*Taking the MCAT Exam.*" AAMC Students, Applicants, and Residents. AAMC, n.d. Web. 2 Dec. 2015. <https://students-residents.aamc.org/applying-medical-school/taking-mcat-exam/>.
20. Dienstag, J. L. (2008). Relevance and rigor in premedical education. *New England Journal of Medicine*, 359(3), 221-224.
21. Muller, D. (2013). Reforming premedical education—out with the old, in with the new. *New England Journal of Medicine*, 368(17), 1567-1569.
22. "*Education and Training: Family Physicians and Nurse Practitioners.*" (n.d.): n. pag. AAFP. Web. 2 Dec. 2015.
23. "MCW-Central Wisconsin." Three Year Discovery Curriculum. Medical College of Wisconsin, 2014. Web. 2 Dec. 2015. <http://www.mcw.edu/Medical-School/Home/Admissions/Central-Wisconsin-Campus.htm>.
24. "FMAT Family Medicine Accelerated Track." Texas Tech University Health Sciences Center School of Medicine, 2015. Web. 02 Dec. 2015. <https://www.ttuhsc.edu/som/fammed/fmat/default.aspx>.
25. "Three-Year MD Pathway." Education and Training. NYU School of Medicine, n.d. Web. 2 Dec. 2015. <http://www.med.nyu.edu/school/student-resources/medical-education/md-curriculum/three-year-md-degree>.
26. "How to Apply: Direct-Entry Masters." Boston College William F. Connell School of Nursing, 13 Nov. 2015. Web. 2 Dec. 2015. <http://www.bc.edu/schools/son/admissions/master_s_entry.html>.
27. "Medical Schools." *Guide - How to Choose a Medical School*. Start Class, 2015. Web. 2 Dec. 2015. <http://medical-schools.startclass.com/>.
28. Squire, L. R. (1989). On the course of forgetting in very long-term memory. *Journal of Experimental Psychology: Learning, Memory, and Cognition*, 15(2), 241.
29. Rohde, Rodney E. "The Hidden Profession That Saves Lives." *Elsevier Connect*. Elsevier, 11 Feb. 2014. Web. 22 June 2015. <http://www.elsevier.com/connect/the-hidden-profession-that-saves-lives>.
30. Hornstein, Lucy, M.D. "Why OB/GYNs Are Not Primary Care Physicians."*Kevin MD, Social Media's Leading Physician Voice*. KevinMD.com, 21 Mar. 2013. Web. 5 Dec. 2015. <http://www.kevinmd.com/blog/2013/03/obgyns-primary-care-physicians.html>.
31. Martin-Misener, R., Harbman, P., Donald, F., Reid, K., Kilpatrick, K., Carter, N., ... & DiCenso, A. (2015). Cost-effectiveness of nurse practitioners in primary and specialised ambulatory care: systematic review. *BMJ open*, 5(6), e007167.
32. Petterson, S. M., Liaw, W. R., Phillips, R. L., Rabin, D. L., Meyers, D. S., & Bazemore, A. W. (2012). Projecting US primary care physician workforce needs: 2010-2025. *The Annals of Family Medicine*, 10(6), 503-509.

33. Jones, D. (2012). Realizing the IOM future of nursing research within clinical practice. *Nursing research*, 61(5), 315.
34. Green, L. V., Savin, S., & Lu, Y. (2013). Primary care physician shortages could be eliminated through use of teams, nonphysicians, and electronic communication. *Health Affairs*, 32(1), 11-19.

Lane 29

Lane 30

www.ingramcontent.com/pod-product-compliance
Lightning Source LLC
Chambersburg PA
CBHW080528190526
45169CB00008B/3097